Juicing for Life: Nourishing Recipes to Support Cancer Patients"

By Eric A. Sherman

Table of contents

Chapter 1. Why juicing is beneficial for cancer patients

Cancer is a devastating disease that can affect anyone at any time. It is a condition that requires extensive treatment, including chemotherapy, radiation, and surgery. In addition to traditional cancer treatments, many patients have turned to alternative therapies to help them cope with the side effects of cancer and its treatments. One of these alternative therapies is juicing.

Juicing is the process of extracting the juice from fruits and vegetables. The juice is often consumed as a beverage, and it can be a quick and convenient way to get essential nutrients into the body. For cancer patients, juicing can be beneficial for several reasons.

Firstly, juicing is an excellent way to consume a wide variety of fruits and vegetables, which are high in vitamins, minerals, and antioxidants. These nutrients are essential for maintaining good health, and they can help the body fight cancer by strengthening the immune system and reducing inflammation. In particular, antioxidants can help protect the body from the damage caused by free radicals, which can contribute to the development of cancer.

Secondly, juicing can be a good way to consume fruits and vegetables that cancer patients may have difficulty eating in their whole form. For example, some patients may experience nausea or difficulty swallowing due to their cancer or treatment. Juicing can provide a way to consume these essential nutrients without causing discomfort.

Thirdly, juicing can help cancer patients maintain their weight and strength during treatment. Cancer treatments can often cause patients to lose weight and muscle mass, which can weaken the body and make it more difficult to recover. Juicing can provide a quick and easy way to consume calories and nutrients to help maintain weight and energy levels.

Finally, juicing can be a great way to help cancer patients stay hydrated. Dehydration can be a common problem for cancer patients, especially those undergoing chemotherapy or radiation. Juicing can provide a quick and easy way to consume fluids and electrolytes to help maintain hydration levels.

It is important to note that juicing should not be used as a replacement for traditional cancer treatments. While juicing can provide many benefits, it is not a cure for cancer. However, it can be an excellent complementary therapy to help cancer patients cope with the side effects of treatment and maintain their health and wellness.

In conclusion, juicing can be a beneficial therapy for cancer patients. It can provide a quick and convenient way to consume essential nutrients, help patients maintain their weight and strength, and keep them hydrated during treatment. If you are a cancer patient considering juicing, it is important to consult with your doctor or a nutritionist to ensure that you are consuming a balanced and healthy diet that meets your specific needs and requirements.

Balanced Diet During Cancer.

The importance of a balanced diet during cancer treatment

Maintaining a balanced diet is important during cancer treatment for several reasons. Firstly, cancer treatments such as chemotherapy, radiation therapy, and surgery can cause a range of side effects that can impact a person's appetite and ability to eat. Some common side effects include nausea, vomiting, mouth sores, taste changes, and fatigue. Eating a balanced diet can help to manage these side effects and maintain strength and energy.

Secondly, a balanced diet can help to support the immune system and help the body to fight off infections and other complications that can occur during cancer treatment. This is particularly important for people with cancer, as they may have a weakened immune system as a result of their treatment.

A balanced diet should include a variety of foods from all food groups, including fruits, vegetables, whole grains, lean proteins, and healthy fats. It is also important to stay hydrated by drinking plenty of water and other fluids.

In addition to a balanced diet, some people with cancer may benefit from working with a registered dietitian who can provide personalized nutrition recommendations and help to manage any side effects or complications related to treatment.

How this cookbook can help cancer patients incorporate healthy juices into their diets

Cookbooks can be a great resource for cancer patients who are looking to incorporate healthy juices into their diets. Here are some ways this cookbook can help:

Provides recipes: The cookbook can provide a variety of recipes for healthy juices that are specifically tailored to meet the nutritional needs of cancer patients. This can include juices that are rich in antioxidants, vitamins, and minerals that can help boost the immune system, promote healing, and reduce inflammation.

Offers guidance on ingredients: The cookbook can provide guidance on choosing ingredients that are safe and beneficial for cancer patients. For example, the cookbook may recommend avoiding certain fruits and vegetables that may interact with cancer treatments, or may suggest using organic produce to avoid exposure to harmful pesticides.

Provides nutritional information: The cookbook can provide nutritional information for each recipe, including the amount of calories, carbohydrates, protein, and fat in each serving. This can be helpful for cancer patients who are trying to maintain a healthy weight or manage specific dietary restrictions.

Offers tips on preparation: The cookbook may offer tips on how to prepare and store juices to maximize their nutritional benefits. For example, the cookbook may suggest using a juicer to extract the most nutrients from fruits and vegetables, or may recommend storing juices in airtight containers to prevent oxidation and nutrient loss.

Provides inspiration and motivation: Finally, the cookbook can provide inspiration and motivation for cancer patients who may be struggling to find healthy and appetizing foods to incorporate into their diets. Seeing a variety of delicious and nutritious juice recipes can help cancer patients feel empowered and motivated to take control of their health and nutrition.

Chapter 2. Juicing Basics

Juicing Basics

Juicing is a method of extracting juice from fruits and vegetables, providing a concentrated source of nutrients in an easy-to-digest form. Here are some basics to get started with juicing:

Choosing a Juicer: There are two main types of juicers - centrifugal and masticating. Centrifugal juicers are typically less expensive and faster, while masticating juicers are slower and more expensive, but can extract more juice and retain more nutrients.

Choosing Ingredients: Use fresh, organic fruits and vegetables whenever possible. Popular ingredients for juicing include leafy greens, apples, carrots, celery, beets, and ginger.

Preparation: Wash your produce thoroughly and cut into small pieces that will fit into your juicer. Remove any inedible parts such as seeds, stems, and pits.

Juicing: Follow the instructions for your specific juicer. Generally, you'll feed the produce into the juicer one piece at a time and collect the juice in a container.

Cleanup: Rinse your juicer parts with warm water immediately after use to prevent buildup. Some parts may be dishwasher safe, but check your manual for specific instructions.

Storing: Juice is best consumed immediately after juicing to maximize nutrient content, but can be stored in an airtight container in the refrigerator for up to 72 hours. If the juice separates, simply stir or shake before consuming.

It's important to note that while juicing can be a healthy addition to your diet, it should not be used as a replacement for whole fruits and vegetables. A balanced diet should still include a variety of whole foods for optimal nutrition.

Types of juicers and their pros and cons

There are three main types of juicers: centrifugal juicers, masticating juicers, and citrus juicers. Here are their pros and cons:

Centrifugal juicers:
Centrifugal juicers are the most common type of juicer, and they work by using a fast-spinning blade to extract juice from fruits and vegetables.

Pros:

Fast and easy to use
Generally more affordable than other types of juicers
Can handle hard fruits and vegetables with ease
Cons:

Less efficient at extracting juice than other types of juicers
Produce more heat, which can lead to oxidation and nutrient loss
Noisy during operation
May not be suitable for juicing leafy greens
Masticating juicers:

Masticating juicers, also known as slow juicers or cold press juicers, use a slow rotating auger to crush and squeeze fruits and vegetables to extract juice.

Pros:

More efficient at extracting juice than centrifugal juicers
Produce less heat, which can lead to less oxidation and nutrient loss
Can juice a wider variety of produce, including leafy greens
Generally produce a higher quality juice with more nutrients and enzymes
Cons:

More expensive than centrifugal juicers
Slower and may require more preparation time
Some models can be difficult to clean
Citrus juicers:
Citrus juicers are designed specifically for juicing citrus fruits like oranges, lemons, and grapefruits.

Pros:

Simple to use and easy to clean
Typically more affordable than other types of juicers

Can extract a high yield of juice from citrus fruits

Cons:

Limited to juicing citrus fruits only

May not be as efficient at extracting juice from other types of produce

May not be suitable for large quantities of juice extraction

Overall, the type of juicer you choose depends on your specific juicing needs and preferences. If you're juicing mostly hard fruits and vegetables, a centrifugal juicer may be a good choice. If you're looking for maximum nutrient extraction and are willing to invest more time and money, a masticating juicer may be a better fit. And if you're only interested in juicing citrus fruits, a citrus juicer is the way to go.

Produce for Juicing

Choosing the best produce for juicing

Choosing the best produce for juicing is an important step to ensure that you get the most out of your juicing experience. Here are some tips to help you select the best produce for juicing:

Look for fresh, ripe produce: Fresh and ripe produce will yield the most juice and provide the best flavor. Choose fruits and vegetables that are firm, without any bruises or soft spots.

Opt for organic: When possible, choose organic produce to avoid exposure to harmful pesticides and chemicals.

Choose a variety of colors: Different colored fruits and vegetables contain different nutrients, so try to choose a variety of colors to ensure that you're getting a range of vitamins and minerals.

Select produce in season: Choosing produce that is in season will often provide the best flavor and nutritional value.

Wash and prep your produce: Before juicing, be sure to wash and prep your produce by removing any stems, seeds, or tough skins. This will help to ensure that you're getting the most juice and nutrients possible.

Some great produce options for juicing include:

Leafy greens like kale, spinach, and collard greens

Citrus fruits like oranges, grapefruits, and lemons

Berries like strawberries, blueberries, and raspberries

Apples and pears

Carrots and beets

Cucumbers and celery

Ginger and turmeric

Remember to experiment with different produce combinations to find the flavor and nutritional profile that works best for you.

Juicing techniques and tips for maximum yield

Juicing is a great way to get essential nutrients and vitamins from fruits and vegetables. Here are some techniques and tips for maximum yield when juicing:

Choose the right produce: Choose fresh, ripe fruits and vegetables with no bruising or soft spots. For maximum yield, go for fruits and vegetables that are naturally high in juice, such as oranges, grapefruits, lemons, cucumbers, and celery.

Prepare your produce: Wash your produce thoroughly before juicing. Remove any pits, seeds, or tough skins from fruits and vegetables that don't juice well, such as apples and carrots.

Use a high-quality juicer: Invest in a good-quality juicer that is capable of extracting the maximum amount of juice from your produce. A masticating or cold press juicer is best for yielding the highest amount of juice.

Juice in batches: To avoid clogging your juicer and to maximize yield, juice your produce in small batches rather than trying to juice all of it at once.

Use a pulp strainer: Using a pulp strainer will help remove any remaining pulp or fibers from your juice, which can increase the amount of juice you can extract.

Juice leafy greens first: If you are juicing leafy greens, juice them first, as they can clog your juicer if you juice them after denser fruits and vegetables.

Alternate produce: Alternate between juicing softer and harder fruits and vegetables, as this can help prevent clogging and maximize yield.

Save the pulp: Don't throw away the pulp left over from juicing. It can be used in a variety of ways, such as adding it to soups, stews, or smoothies.

Drink immediately: Freshly juiced fruits and vegetables are best consumed immediately after juicing to maximize their nutritional value.

By following these techniques and tips, you can maximize the amount of juice you extract from your fruits and vegetables, and enjoy the health benefits of fresh, nutrient-rich juice.

Storing and preserving juice

Storing and preserving juice can be done in a few different ways, depending on the type of juice and how long you want to store it.

Refrigeration: Most juices can be stored in the refrigerator for a few days to a week. Make sure the juice is in an airtight container to prevent oxidation and loss of flavor. Some juices, like freshly squeezed citrus juices, can be stored in the refrigerator for up to two weeks.

Freezing: Juices can also be frozen to preserve them for longer periods of time. Pour the juice into an airtight container, leaving some room at the top for expansion as the juice freezes. When you're ready to use the juice, thaw it in the refrigerator or at room temperature.

Canning: If you want to preserve juice for even longer, you can can it. This involves heating the juice to a high temperature to kill bacteria, then sealing it in jars. Canned juice can last for up to a year or more.

Pasteurization: Commercially sold juices are often pasteurized to kill bacteria and increase shelf life. This involves heating the juice to a high temperature for a short period of time, then quickly cooling it. Pasteurized juices can be stored at room temperature for several months.

Regardless of how you store your juice, it's important to keep it away from light and heat, which can cause it to spoil more quickly. And always check for signs of spoilage, like a sour smell or off taste, before consuming.

Chapter 3.Nutrition for Cancer Patients

Cancer patients require optimal nutrition to maintain their health, support their immune system, and promote healing. However, the disease and its treatment can often lead to loss of appetite, difficulty swallowing, nausea, vomiting, and changes in taste and smell. These issues can make it challenging for cancer patients to get the nutrients they need, which is why understanding their nutritional needs is crucial.

Macronutrients

Cancer patients require adequate amounts of macronutrients, including carbohydrates, proteins, and fats.

Carbohydrates provide energy and should make up 45-65% of the patient's caloric intake. Foods such as fruits, vegetables, whole grains, and legumes are excellent sources of carbohydrates.

Proteins are essential for building and repairing tissues, maintaining immune function, and producing enzymes and hormones. Cancer patients require more protein than healthy individuals, as their bodies need to repair damaged tissues and support immune function. Protein sources such as lean meats, poultry, fish, eggs, dairy products, legumes, and nuts are excellent choices.

Fats are important for energy, absorption of fat-soluble vitamins, and hormone production. It is recommended that cancer patients consume healthy fats such as monounsaturated and polyunsaturated fats found in foods such as nuts, seeds, avocado, and fatty fish.

Micronutrients

Cancer patients also require adequate amounts of micronutrients, including vitamins and minerals, to maintain their health. Some of the essential micronutrients that cancer patients need include:

Vitamin D: Vitamin D is essential for maintaining bone health and promoting immune function. Cancer patients may be at risk of vitamin D deficiency due to limited sun exposure and lack of appetite. Foods such as fatty fish, egg yolks, and fortified dairy products are good sources of vitamin D.

Vitamin C: Vitamin C is important for immune function and wound healing. It is also an antioxidant that protects cells from damage. Foods such as citrus fruits, berries, kiwi, and broccoli are excellent sources of vitamin C.

Vitamin E: Vitamin E is an antioxidant that protects cells from damage and promotes immune function. It is found in foods such as nuts, seeds, vegetable oils, and leafy green vegetables.

Iron: Iron is essential for the production of red blood cells, which carry oxygen throughout the body. Cancer patients may be at risk of iron deficiency due to chemotherapy-induced anemia. Foods such as red meat, poultry, fish, beans, and fortified cereals are good sources of iron.

Calcium: Calcium is essential for maintaining strong bones and teeth. Cancer patients may be at risk of calcium deficiency due to lack of appetite and reduced intake of dairy products. Foods such as dairy products, leafy green vegetables, and fortified cereals are good sources of calcium.

Fluids

Cancer patients may experience dehydration due to vomiting, diarrhea, or decreased fluid intake. It is essential to drink adequate amounts of fluids to maintain hydration and prevent complications such as kidney failure. Patients should aim to drink at least eight cups of fluid per day, including water, tea, soup, and juice.

Conclusion

Cancer patients require adequate nutrition to maintain their health, promote healing, and support immune function. It is essential to consume a balanced diet that includes macronutrients, micronutrients, and fluids. Patients may benefit from working with a registered dietitian who can provide personalized nutrition recommendations based on their individual needs and treatment plan. A healthy diet can help cancer patients maintain their strength, reduce the risk of complications, and improve their quality of life.

Chapter 4.Cancer Treatment Nutrition Impact

Overview of cancer treatment and its impact on nutrition

Cancer treatment refers to the various methods used to treat cancer, including surgery, chemotherapy, radiation therapy, immunotherapy, targeted therapy, and hormone therapy. While these treatments can be effective in fighting cancer, they can also have a significant impact on a person's nutritional status.

Chemotherapy and radiation therapy can cause side effects such as nausea, vomiting, diarrhea, and loss of appetite, which can lead to malnutrition. These treatments can also cause changes in taste and smell, making it difficult to enjoy food. Surgery can also cause changes in the digestive system that can affect the way nutrients are absorbed.

Furthermore, cancer itself can cause changes in the body's metabolism, leading to weight loss, muscle wasting, and malnutrition. This can further exacerbate the impact of cancer treatment on nutrition.

As a result, it is important for cancer patients to receive appropriate nutrition support throughout their treatment. This may include working with a registered dietitian to develop an individualized nutrition plan that meets their needs and preferences, as well as addressing any specific side effects or challenges related to their treatment.

Nutrition support may include oral nutrition supplements, enteral nutrition (feeding through a tube), or parenteral nutrition (feeding through an IV). It may also involve modifying the texture or composition of food to make it easier to tolerate or absorb.

In addition to improving overall nutrition status, adequate nutrition can also help reduce treatment-related side effects, improve immune function, and enhance quality of life for cancer patients. Therefore, nutrition should be an integral part of cancer treatment and care.

Essential nutrients for cancer patients

Cancer patients have unique nutritional needs due to the impact of cancer and its treatments on the body. Eating a balanced and nutritious diet is essential to maintain strength, prevent infections, and promote recovery during and after cancer treatment. Here are some essential nutrients for cancer patients:

Protein: Protein is essential for repairing and building tissues, maintaining immune function, and preventing muscle loss. Cancer patients may need more protein than healthy individuals to support their body's needs. Good sources of protein include lean meats, poultry, fish, eggs, beans, nuts, and dairy products.

Fiber: Fiber helps to regulate bowel movements and prevent constipation, which can be a side effect of cancer treatments. It also helps to maintain healthy blood sugar levels and prevent weight gain. Good sources of fiber include whole grains, fruits, vegetables, beans, and nuts.

Vitamins and minerals: Cancer patients may need additional vitamins and minerals to support their immune system and prevent nutrient deficiencies. Good sources of vitamins and minerals include fruits, vegetables, whole grains, and lean meats.

Omega-3 fatty acids: Omega-3 fatty acids have anti-inflammatory properties and may help to reduce inflammation and improve immune function. Good sources of omega-3 fatty acids include fatty fish, such as salmon and tuna, flaxseeds, chia seeds, and walnuts.

Water: Drinking plenty of water is essential for staying hydrated, preventing constipation, and flushing toxins out of the body. Cancer patients should aim to drink at least eight cups of water per day, and more if they are experiencing diarrhea or vomiting.

It is important for cancer patients to work with their healthcare team, including a registered dietitian, to develop an individualized nutrition plan that meets their unique needs and preferences.

How juicing can help meet nutritional needs

Juicing can be an excellent way to meet your nutritional needs. By using a juicer to extract the juice from fruits and vegetables, you can consume a concentrated source of vitamins, minerals, and other essential nutrients.

One of the primary benefits of juicing is that it allows you to consume a large amount of produce quickly and easily. Many people find it challenging to consume the recommended daily servings of fruits and vegetables, but juicing can make it easier to meet those requirements. For example, you could easily consume several servings of leafy greens, carrots, and other produce in a single glass of juice.

Juicing can also be an effective way to get more nutrients from certain fruits and vegetables. Some plant foods, such as leafy greens, can be challenging to digest, making it difficult for your body to extract all the nutrients. Juicing breaks down the cell walls of these foods, making the nutrients more accessible to your body.

Furthermore, juicing can be an excellent way to boost your intake of specific nutrients that you may be lacking. For example, if you're not getting enough vitamin C, juicing citrus fruits can help you meet your needs. Juicing can also be a great way to consume more antioxidants, which are essential for fighting inflammation and protecting against chronic disease.

However, it's important to note that juicing should not be your sole source of nutrition. While juicing can be a healthy addition to your diet, it's important to continue to consume whole fruits and vegetables as well. Whole produce contains fiber, which is essential for digestive health, and can help you feel full and satisfied.

In summary, juicing can be a great way to meet your nutritional needs by providing a concentrated source of vitamins, minerals, and other essential nutrients. However, it should be used in conjunction with a balanced diet that includes a variety of whole fruits and vegetables.

Chapter 5.Juicing Recipes.

Juicing Recipes

Here are three different juicing recipes you can try:

Green Juice:

1 green apple

1 cucumber

2 cups of spinach

1 lemon

1 knob of ginger

1 handful of parsley

Carrot-Orange Juice:

4-5 large carrots

2 oranges

1-inch piece of ginger

Beetroot-Apple Juice:

2 medium-sized beetroots

2 green apples

1 large cucumber

1-inch piece of ginger

Instructions:

Wash and chop all the ingredients into smaller pieces to fit in the juicer.

Feed the ingredients through the juicer.

Serve immediately or store in an airtight container in the fridge for up to 24 hours.

Note: Always consult with your doctor or a nutritionist if you have any underlying health conditions or if you are pregnant or breastfeeding before making any changes to your diet.

Apple Ginger Juice Recipe

Apple and ginger juice
Apple and ginger juice is a delicious and healthy drink that can be made by combining fresh apples and ginger root in a juicer or blender. Here's a simple recipe to make apple and ginger juice:

Ingredients:

2 medium-sized apples, cored and chopped
1 inch piece of fresh ginger root, peeled and chopped

1 cup of water (optional)

Instructions:

Wash the apples and ginger root thoroughly.

Cut the apples into small pieces and remove the core.

Peel and chop the ginger root into small pieces.

Add the chopped apples and ginger to a juicer or blender.

If using a blender, add one cup of water.

Blend or juice the mixture until it is smooth and well combined.

Strain the juice through a fine mesh strainer or cheesecloth to remove any pulp or fibers.

Serve the juice immediately over ice or store it in the refrigerator for up to 2 days.

Enjoy your refreshing and healthy apple and ginger juice!

Pineapple Turmeric Juice

Pineapple and turmeric juice

Pineapple and turmeric juice is a popular health drink that is believed to offer a range of health benefits. Pineapple is rich in vitamins C and B6, as well as minerals like potassium and manganese. It also contains an enzyme called bromelain, which has anti-inflammatory properties. Turmeric, on the other hand, contains curcumin, a powerful antioxidant that has anti-inflammatory and anti-cancer properties.

To make pineapple and turmeric juice, you will need the following ingredients:

1 cup of fresh pineapple chunks
1 teaspoon of turmeric powder
1/2 cup of water
1 tablespoon of honey (optional)
Here are the steps to follow:

Add the pineapple chunks and turmeric powder to a blender.
Add water and blend until smooth.
Taste the juice and add honey if you prefer a sweeter taste.
Serve the juice immediately, or refrigerate for later use.
Pineapple and turmeric juice is best consumed fresh and can be consumed as part of a healthy and balanced diet. However, if you have any health concerns or are taking any medication, it is important to consult with your healthcare provider before adding this juice to your diet.

Blueberry Beetroot Juice Recipe.

Blueberry and beetroot juice:
Blueberry and beetroot juice is a delicious and nutritious drink that combines the natural sweetness of blueberries with the earthy flavor of beetroots. Here's a simple recipe for making this juice:

Ingredients:

1 cup of blueberries
1 medium-sized beetroot
1/2 cup of water
Instructions:

Wash and clean the blueberries and beetroot.

Peel the beetroot and chop it into small pieces.

Add the blueberries and chopped beetroot into a blender.

Add half a cup of water into the blender.

Blend the ingredients together until they form a smooth juice.

Strain the juice through a fine mesh strainer to remove any pulp or chunks.

Serve the juice in a glass and enjoy!

Blueberry and beetroot juice is rich in antioxidants, vitamins, and minerals that are beneficial for your health. It can help boost your immune system, improve your digestion, and provide a natural energy boost.

Vegetable-based juices:

Carrot-Kale Juice Preparations.

Carrot and kale juice preparations:
Carrot and kale juice is a delicious and nutritious way to start your day. Here are two different ways to prepare this tasty juice:

Carrot and Kale Juice with Lemon
Ingredients:

2 large carrots, washed and peeled
2 cups kale, washed and chopped
1 lemon, juiced
1 inch piece of ginger, peeled
1 cup water
Instructions:

Add the carrots, kale, ginger, and water to a blender and blend until smooth.

Strain the mixture through a fine mesh sieve or cheesecloth to remove any pulp.

Stir in the lemon juice and serve immediately.

Carrot and Kale Juice with Apple

Ingredients:

2 large carrots, washed and peeled
2 cups kale, washed and chopped

1 apple, cored and sliced
1/2 cucumber, peeled and sliced
1/2 lemon, juiced
Instructions:

Add the carrots, kale, apple, cucumber, and lemon juice to a juicer and process according to the manufacturer's instructions.
Serve immediately over ice.
Both of these recipes are delicious and nutritious ways to enjoy carrot and kale juice. Try them both and see which one you like best!

Spinach Cucumber Juice.

Spinach and cucumber juice:
Spinach and cucumber juice is a refreshing and healthy beverage that can be enjoyed any time of the day. Here's how you can make it:

Ingredients:

1 cucumber
2 cups spinach leaves

1/2 lemon, juiced

1/2 inch piece of ginger

1/4 cup water

Instructions:

Wash the cucumber and spinach leaves thoroughly.

Peel the cucumber if desired, then cut it into chunks.

Add the cucumber chunks, spinach leaves, lemon juice, and ginger to a blender.

Blend until the mixture is smooth and well-combined.

If the mixture is too thick, add water to thin it out to your desired consistency.

Pour the juice into a glass and enjoy immediately.

This juice is a great way to get your daily dose of vegetables and is packed with vitamins and minerals that are essential for good health. It's also a low-calorie beverage that can help you stay hydrated throughout the day.

Broccoli Ginger Juice Recipe.

Broccoli and ginger juice:
Broccoli and ginger juice is a nutritious and flavorful drink that can provide many health benefits. Here's a simple recipe you can try at home:

Ingredients:

2 cups broccoli florets
1 inch piece of fresh ginger, peeled and chopped
1 apple, cored and chopped
1 lemon, juiced
1 cup water
Instructions:

Wash the broccoli and chop it into small florets.
Peel and chop the ginger.
Core and chop the apple.
Add the broccoli, ginger, apple, and water to a blender.
Blend until smooth.

Strain the mixture through a fine mesh strainer.

Stir in the lemon juice.

Pour the juice into a glass and enjoy!

This juice is a great way to consume more vegetables, as broccoli is packed with vitamins and minerals. Ginger is known for its anti-inflammatory properties, while lemon provides a boost of vitamin C. The apple adds sweetness and helps to balance out the flavors. Enjoy!

Nutrient-dense juices

Wheatgrass and ginger shots.

Wheatgrass and ginger shot juice preparations:

Wheatgrass and ginger shot juice preparations are both popular health drinks that are believed to offer a range of health benefits. Here are some possible ways to prepare these shots:

Wheatgrass Shot:

Ingredients:

1-2 oz of fresh wheatgrass juice

1 oz of lemon juice

1 tsp of honey

Instructions:

Rinse the wheatgrass thoroughly under running water.

Cut the wheatgrass into small pieces and juice it using a wheatgrass juicer.

Mix the wheatgrass juice with lemon juice and honey.

Stir the mixture well.

Drink immediately.

Ginger Shot:

Ingredients:

1 oz of fresh ginger juice

1 oz of lemon juice

1 tsp of honey

1 pinch of cayenne pepper

Instructions:

Peel and grate fresh ginger.

Squeeze the grated ginger using a cheesecloth or juicer to obtain 1 oz of ginger juice.

Mix ginger juice, lemon juice, honey, and cayenne pepper in a shot glass.

Stir well.

Drink immediately.

Note: The taste of both wheatgrass and ginger shots can be quite strong, so it may take some getting used to. It's also a good idea to start with small amounts and gradually increase the dose as you get used to the taste and effects. Additionally, these shots are not suitable for everyone, so be sure to consult with your doctor before trying them.

Spirulina Pineapple Juice

Spirulina and pineapple juice preparations:

Spirulina is a type of blue-green algae that is often marketed as a dietary supplement due to its high protein and nutrient content. Pineapple juice is a juice made from the fruit of the pineapple plant.

There are a variety of ways to prepare spirulina and pineapple juice, but one popular method is to blend the two together to create a nutritious and refreshing beverage. Here's a simple recipe to try:

Ingredients:

1 cup pineapple juice
1 tsp spirulina powder
Instructions:

Add the pineapple juice and spirulina powder to a blender.
Blend on high until the spirulina is fully incorporated and
the mixture is smooth.
Pour the mixture into a glass and enjoy!
Note that the flavor of spirulina can be quite strong and
earthy, so you may want to adjust the amount of spirulina to
taste. Some people also like to add other ingredients to the
mix, such as bananas, honey, or coconut water, for added
flavor and nutrition.

Sweet potato carrot juice.

Sweet potato and carrot juice preparations:

Sweet potato and carrot juice is a healthy and delicious drink
that is rich in nutrients, vitamins, and minerals. Here are
two simple recipes for sweet potato and carrot juice:

Recipe 1: Sweet Potato and Carrot Juice

Ingredients:

1 sweet potato, peeled and chopped
2 carrots, peeled and chopped
1/2 inch ginger, peeled and grated
1 apple, cored and chopped
1 cup water
Instructions:

In a blender or juicer, combine the sweet potato, carrots, ginger, apple, and water.
Blend or juice until smooth.
Pour the juice into a glass and serve.
Recipe 2: Spiced Sweet Potato and Carrot Juice

Ingredients:

1 sweet potato, peeled and chopped
2 carrots, peeled and chopped
1/2 inch ginger, peeled and grated
1/2 teaspoon ground cinnamon
1/4 teaspoon ground nutmeg

1/4 teaspoon ground cloves

1 cup water

Instructions:

In a blender or juicer, combine the sweet potato, carrots, ginger, cinnamon, nutmeg, cloves, and water.

Blend or juice until smooth.

Pour the juice into a glass and serve.

Both of these recipes make one serving of sweet potato and carrot juice. You can adjust the amount of water based on how thick or thin you prefer your juice. Enjoy!

Chapter 6. Meal Planning with Juices

Juice Meal Planning.

Meal Planning with Juices:
Meal planning with juices can be a fun and healthy way to incorporate more fruits and vegetables into your diet. Here are some tips for incorporating juices into your meal plan:

Choose a variety of fruits and vegetables: Juicing allows you to consume a larger variety of fruits and vegetables than you may typically eat in a day. Choose a range of colors and textures to get a diverse array of nutrients.

Consider nutrient balance: While it's tempting to stick to fruit juices, try to balance your intake of fruits and vegetables. Vegetables are typically lower in sugar and higher in nutrients like fiber, vitamins, and minerals.

Pair juices with meals: Consider pairing your juice with a meal or snack. For example, a green juice with leafy greens, cucumber, and lemon could be a refreshing addition to a salad or wrap.

Plan ahead: Consider prepping your fruits and vegetables ahead of time, so you can quickly whip up a juice when you need it. You can also freeze pre-cut fruits and veggies for later use.

Get creative: Don't be afraid to experiment with different flavors and combinations. Adding ginger, turmeric, or fresh herbs like mint can give your juices a unique flavor and added health benefits.

Here's an example of a meal plan incorporating juices:

Breakfast: Green smoothie with spinach, banana, almond milk, and a scoop of protein powder.

Snack: Carrot and ginger juice.

Lunch: Quinoa and vegetable salad with a side of fresh orange juice.

Snack: Beet, apple, and ginger juice.

Dinner: Grilled salmon with a side of roasted vegetables and a green juice with kale, cucumber, and lemon.

Dessert: Berry and avocado smoothie with almond milk.

Incorporating juices into meals

Incorporating juices into meals can be a great way to add flavor, nutrition, and variety to your diet. Here are some ideas for how to incorporate juices into your meals:

Smoothies: Smoothies are a great way to incorporate juices into your breakfast or snack. You can use any type of juice as a base and add fruits, vegetables, nuts, and seeds to make a delicious and nutritious smoothie.

Salad dressings: Use fruit juices like orange or pomegranate juice to make a tasty and healthy salad dressing. Mix the juice with olive oil, vinegar, and spices to make a tangy dressing that will add a pop of flavor to your salads.

Marinades: Use citrus juices like lemon or lime juice to make a flavorful marinade for meats or tofu. The acidity of the juice will help to tenderize the protein and infuse it with delicious flavor.

Sauces: Use vegetable juices like carrot or tomato juice to make a tasty sauce for pasta, rice, or vegetables. You can also use fruit juices like apple or cranberry juice to make a sweet and tangy sauce for desserts.

Soups: Use vegetable juices like tomato or carrot juice as a base for your soups. Add herbs, spices, and other vegetables to create a hearty and nutritious soup that will warm you up on a cold day.

By incorporating juices into your meals, you can add a variety of flavors and nutrients to your diet. Just be sure to choose juices that are low in added sugars and high in vitamins and minerals.

Juicing for All Meals

Juicing for breakfast, lunch, and dinner

Juicing for all three meals of the day may not be a balanced and sustainable approach to nutrition. While juicing can provide some benefits, such as a quick and easy way to consume fruits and vegetables, it is important to consider the potential drawbacks.

One concern is that juicing removes the fiber from fruits and vegetables, which can lead to a rapid spike in blood sugar levels. This can cause energy crashes and hunger pangs soon after drinking the juice, which may lead to overeating or choosing less healthy food options later in the day.

In addition, relying solely on juices for meals can result in a lack of essential nutrients such as protein, healthy fats, and complex carbohydrates, which are necessary for maintaining energy levels, building and repairing tissues, and supporting overall health.

While incorporating fresh juices into a healthy diet can be a good idea, it is important to balance them with other nutritious whole foods to ensure you are getting all the nutrients your body needs. Consulting a registered dietitian or healthcare professional can help you determine the best approach for your individual needs and goals.

Juices with Healthy Snacks

Pairing juices with healthy snacks:

Pairing juices with healthy snacks is a great way to ensure that you are getting the nutrition you need to support a healthy lifestyle. Here are a few ideas for pairing juices with healthy snacks:

Carrot juice with hummus and vegetables: Carrot juice is high in vitamin A and antioxidants, which are essential for healthy skin and a strong immune system. Pair it with hummus and a variety of fresh vegetables like cucumbers, carrots, and bell peppers for a satisfying and nutritious snack.

Apple juice with almond butter and apple slices: Apple juice is a good source of vitamin C and antioxidants, which can help protect your cells from damage. Pair it with almond butter and apple slices for a snack that is high in fiber and protein.

Beet juice with roasted chickpeas: Beet juice is rich in nitrates, which can help improve blood flow and reduce blood pressure. Pair it with roasted chickpeas for a snack that is high in protein, fiber, and healthy fats.

Orange juice with Greek yogurt and berries: Orange juice is high in vitamin C and other antioxidants, which can help boost your immune system. Pair it with Greek yogurt and a variety of fresh berries for a snack that is high in protein and fiber.

Remember to choose juices that are low in added sugars and pair them with snacks that are low in processed ingredients and high in nutrients to maximize the health benefits of your snack.

Encouragement to incorporate juicing into daily routines:

Juicing can be a great way to incorporate more fruits and vegetables into your daily routine, and it can provide many health benefits. Here are some tips and encouragement for incorporating juicing into your daily routine:

Start small: If you are new to juicing, start with a small serving size and work your way up. This will help your body adjust to the new nutrients and prevent any digestive discomfort.

Experiment with different ingredients: Try out different combinations of fruits and vegetables to find your favorite flavor. You can also add herbs and spices to give your juice an extra boost of flavor.

Plan ahead: To make juicing a part of your daily routine, it helps to plan ahead. Wash and prep your fruits and vegetables ahead of time so that you can quickly make a juice in the morning or whenever you have a few spare minutes.

Invest in a good juicer: A high-quality juicer can make the process of juicing much easier and more enjoyable. Look for a juicer that is easy to clean and can handle a variety of fruits and vegetables.

Set realistic goals: If you want to incorporate juicing into your daily routine, start with a goal of making one juice a day. As you become more comfortable with juicing, you can increase your goal to two or more juices per day.

Remember, juicing should not replace whole fruits and vegetables in your diet, but it can be a great supplement to help you reach your daily intake of vitamins and minerals. With a little planning and experimentation, incorporating juicing into your daily routine can be a fun and healthy habit to develop.